Transfer your
GIFTS AND PLANS

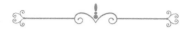

Same Aim - Revised Setting

Dedorah S. Brown

WESTBOW
PRESS®
A DIVISION OF THOMAS NELSON
& ZONDERVAN

WestBow Press books may be ordered through booksellers or by contacting:

WestBow Press
A Division of Thomas Nelson & Zondervan
1663 Liberty Drive
Bloomington, IN 47403
www.westbowpress.com
844-714-3454

ISBN: 979-8-3850-4017-9 (sc)
ISBN: 979-8-3850-4018-6 (e)

Library of Congress Control Number: 2024926505

Print information available on the last page.

WestBow Press rev. date: 01/25/2025

Dedicated to Mr. Kevin G. Brown

Acknowledgments

Thank you to those who were able to teach me life lasting lessons through your actions far beyond your words ever could and special thanks to those service members who served and trained by my side.

Introduction

It is so powerful when you realize your gifts and talents. There is such an awakening when strong feelings arise and tug at your heartstrings causing you to devise a plan so that you can do the things that you envisioned. There are not too many things that can compare to that type of excitement radiating throughout your being. So the decision has been made. You know what you want to do, how you want to go about doing it, when you want to start, the locations where you want to do it and who you want to collaborate with while doing it.

Your plans sound solid and your plans look solid. So you start making moves according to your well-orchestrated plan but something interrupts your flow. Now you are a little thrown off because it seems as if your whole plan has collapsed but that can be challenged if you are up to it. Give yourself the grace that you deserve. Things may not have worked out in that setting but you can transfer your gifts and plans to a more suitable scene. Allow yourself to recognize the dissatisfaction that you feel, pray about it, analyze if it is still worth it to you to continue pursing it then make your move. Please allow me to share three times in my life when I decided that my gifts were worth using and my plans were worth executing so I revised them instead of discording them.

When I was a young girl I wanted to join a dance team. I wanted to join because I loved dancing and because I wanted to participate with the team during our football team's halftime show. I tried out for the squad and according to the moderator and present members I did the routine correctly and with ease. A few of the other girls who were trying out was having a difficult time executing the moves. The moderator asked me to assist them and I was happy to.

The next day there was a list placed on the door of the classroom where the tryouts were held naming those who were selected. I was not selected. I was not happy but I understood that not everyone could be chosen. Later that day while walking home two of the girls who were already a part of that dance team congratulated me for doing so well. Then they went on to say that the only reason why I was not selected was because they had already selected someone that was my height and skin complexion. That was shocking to hear. I did what was within my control during the tryout process but the selection process was out of my control. A few days later I tried out for another dance team and I made the squad. I am saying this with all honesty, this squad was a better fit for my gift and I was still able to participate as a dancer during our football halftime shows. Look at God!

My next testimony started during my early 20's. I was a full-time college student and my plans were to complete my 4 year program in no more than 4 years. During my enrollment I experienced several hardships that contributed to me deciding to dropout and join the military. After serving 10 years of active duty in the United States Army, I immediately returned back to that same university, completed my studies and proudly graduated. In addition to that, I continued on to graduate school and knocked that out as well. My plan was to become a college graduate and although my plans were revised they were not terminated.

My last short story is about my quest to work in the field of social work. I had the education that was necessary for it, I had the skills to do it proficiently, and I had the heart to properly serve those who were assigned to my care. A few short years into the profession I had a few medical examinations that revealed that some of my military experiences altered my health. This ultimately changed my ability to work as I planned. That was something to come to terms with but I refused to let those circumstances stop me from being a lifetime active contributor in as many human improvement endeavors that I was willing to. I am still doing social services but as a wellness influencer, an author of several wellness and behavioral books, an advocate, a speaker, a philanthropist and doing way more than I could working under someone else's mission statement. I am continuing to transfer my gifts and plans by using the same aim but in revised settings while being blessed to see doors fly open for me.

If something has interrupted your plans pray about how you want to proceed, think about how you want to proceed, control what you can control and make your move. Please allow this journaling workbook to assist you on your journey.

Transfer Your Gifts and Plans

Same Aim-Revised Setting

1

Be clear about what you are going after.

Revise Your Plan

_____

_____

_____

_____

_____

_____

_____

_____

_____

_____

2

You are designed to complete your purpose so go ahead and make the product that you were gifted to produce.

Revise Your Plan

_____

_____

_____

_____

_____

_____

_____

_____

_____

_____

3

There will be times when people will enter your life and times when they will leave but you must continue easing on down the road.

Revise Your Plan

_____

_____

_____

_____

_____

_____

_____

_____

_____

_____

4

The direction that you had in mind might have changed its course but it does not mean that you have changed what you had in mind.

Revise Your Plan

_____

_____

_____

_____

_____

_____

_____

_____

_____

_____

5

Sometimes doing what is right may cause you to be
disqualified from things that you are qualified for.

Revise Your Plan

_____

_____

_____

_____

_____

_____

_____

_____

_____

_____

6

Not gaining what you want can at times surprisingly
grant you with something that you really need.

Revise Your Plan

_____

_____

_____

_____

_____

_____

_____

_____

_____

_____

7

It is not worth pleading for a relationship to continue when it is clear that it is damaging your growth.

Revise Your Plan

_____

_____

_____

_____

_____

_____

_____

_____

_____

_____

8

Say farewell to distractions and do right by yourself.

Revise Your Plan

_____

_____

_____

_____

_____

_____

_____

_____

_____

_____

9

Saying yes to things that you honestly know are
not in your best interest is not worth it.

Revise Your Plan

_____

_____

_____

_____

_____

_____

_____

_____

_____

_____

10

When you see people distancing themselves that actually allows more space and privacy to do you.

Revise Your Plan

_____

_____

_____

_____

_____

_____

_____

_____

_____

_____

11

Place your current state of mind in a better state of being so that clearance is made for future endeavors.

Revise Your Plan

_____

_____

_____

_____

_____

_____

_____

_____

_____

_____

12

Some of the denials that you received were not cruel just necessary for how you needed to be developed.

Revise Your Plan

_____

_____

_____

_____

_____

_____

_____

_____

_____

_____

_____

13

Your journey is just for you, your gifts and your plans.

Revise Your Plan

_____

_____

_____

_____

_____

_____

_____

_____

_____

_____

14

If you keep some of the promises that you make with yourself you will be impressed with your results.

Revise Your Plan

_____

_____

_____

_____

_____

_____

_____

_____

_____

_____

15

Try not to give too much attention to what did not work out.

Revise Your Plan

_____

_____

_____

_____

_____

_____

_____

_____

_____

_____

16

Rely more on your prayers than on your prayer partners.

Revise Your Plan

_____

_____

_____

_____

_____

_____

_____

_____

_____

_____

17

Abandoning your quest to jump on board with
someone else's may not work in your favor.

Revise Your Plan

_____

_____

_____

_____

_____

_____

_____

_____

_____

_____

18

If you want to feel empowered and a sense of
accomplishment complete at least one of your goals.

Revise Your Plan

_____

_____

_____

_____

_____

_____

_____

_____

_____

19

Mind your manners with your well-being.

Revise Your Plan

_____

_____

_____

_____

_____

_____

_____

_____

_____

_____

20

When you are not selected for certain settings
your next move might be more fulfilling.

Revise Your Plan

_____

_____

_____

_____

_____

_____

_____

_____

_____

21

Be assured that you are worthy of the gift that you possess.

Revise Your Plan

_____

_____

_____

_____

_____

_____

_____

_____

_____

_____

22

Take your dreams and do something tremendous with them.

Revise Your Plan

_____

_____

_____

_____

_____

_____

_____

_____

_____

23

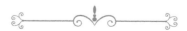

When you walk away from a space that you really wanted to be in but realize that something about it was not right takes some of the sting off.

Revise Your Plan

_____

_____

_____

_____

_____

_____

_____

_____

_____

_____

24

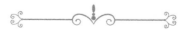

Beware of the fake signals that your heart
and mind sometimes tries to tell you about
why things did not go your way.

Revise Your Plan

_____

_____

_____

_____

_____

_____

_____

_____

_____

25

When you refuse to be at someone's beck and call they
might say that you did not want to play nice when
the truth is you simply did not wish to be played.

Revise Your Plan

_____

_____

_____

_____

_____

_____

_____

_____

_____

_____

26

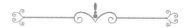

When you change the way that you move and
respond to things you may lose the interest
of some of your peers and family.

Revise Your Plan

_____

_____

_____

_____

_____

_____

_____

_____

_____

_____

27

Neglecting what you need to do for yourself in hopes
of being liked by others will not enhance your gifts.

Revise Your Plan

28

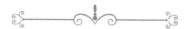

It is good to share but some things should be just for you.

Revise Your Plan

_____

_____

_____

_____

_____

_____

_____

_____

_____

_____

29

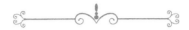

When you are clear that it is time to change
the scene start making necessary moves.

Revise Your Plan

_____

_____

_____

_____

_____

_____

_____

_____

_____

_____

_____

30

It is such a good feeling when you realize that you
have so many gifts sitting before you that it can
be difficult deciding which gift to utilize first.

Revise Your Plan

_____

_____

_____

_____

_____

_____

_____

_____

_____

_____

31

Just because something is popular does not
mean that you should gravitate to it.

Revise Your Plan

_____

_____

_____

_____

_____

_____

_____

_____

_____

32

Not being selected will not leave you depleted but
it will give you another tool to build with.

Revise Your Plan

33

Taking on another person's mannerisms will
diminish your identity so leave that alone.

Revise Your Plan

_____

_____

_____

_____

_____

_____

_____

_____

_____

34

Do not underestimate all of the success that
you can obtain by putting in more effort.

Revise Your Plan

_____

_____

_____

_____

_____

_____

_____

_____

_____

35

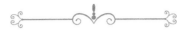

Some of the things that caused you to pause also caused you to draw strength from your stash spot!

Revise Your Plan

_____

_____

_____

_____

_____

_____

_____

_____

_____

36

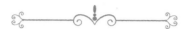

Abolish the energy that keeps you captive
and embrace the energy that throws confetti
over your head in celebration of you!

Revise Your Plan

_____

_____

_____

_____

_____

_____

_____

_____

_____

_____

37

Shine high beam lights on all of your achievements.

Revise Your Plan

_____

_____

_____

_____

_____

_____

_____

_____

_____

38

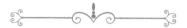

You can hold yourself accountable
without putting yourself down.

Revise Your Plan

_____

_____

_____

_____

_____

_____

_____

_____

_____

_____

39

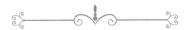

When you fall short just try again.

Revise Your Plan

_____

_____

_____

_____

_____

_____

_____

_____

_____

_____

40

Losing one environment can guide you to the
space where your dreams and ideas reside.

Revise Your Plan

_____

_____

_____

_____

_____

_____

_____

_____

_____

_____

41

At times you can be your own worst enemy so there is no need to hold auditions or interviews for more enemies.

Revise Your Plan

_____

_____

_____

_____

_____

_____

_____

_____

_____

_____

42

Make sure that the action that you take is what you want and not just because someone who you respect suggested it.

Revise Your Plan

_____

_____

_____

_____

_____

_____

_____

_____

_____

_____

43

If you believe that your dreams and ideas
are worth going after then go for it.

Revise Your Plan

_____

_____

_____

_____

_____

_____

_____

_____

_____

_____

44

Keep moving towards your game changing opportunity.

Revise Your Plan

_____

_____

_____

_____

_____

_____

_____

_____

_____

_____

45

Live a lifestyle that allows you to maintain peace.

Revise Your Plan

_____

_____

_____

_____

_____

_____

_____

_____

_____

46

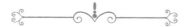

Get educated about what it may take
to get the life that you long for.

Revise Your Plan

_____

_____

_____

_____

_____

_____

_____

_____

_____

47

The reaction that you give can make a situation
worse than it needs to be so watch yourself.

Revise Your Plan

_____

_____

_____

_____

_____

_____

_____

_____

_____

_____

48

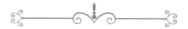

Having to make revisions to your plan is not necessarily a bad thing.

Revise Your Plan

_____

_____

_____

_____

_____

_____

_____

_____

_____

_____

49

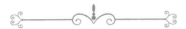

You will have the energy needed to do the
things that you were gifted to do.

Revise Your Plan

_____

_____

_____

_____

_____

_____

_____

_____

_____

_____

50

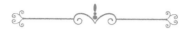

Take care of the unique gifts that
you have been blessed with.

Revise Your Plan

_____

_____

_____

_____

_____

_____

_____

_____

_____

51

Decide on which dreams that you will
go after and devise your plans.

Revise Your Plan

52

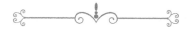

Things do not have to go according to the
original plan in order to be manifested.

Revise Your Plan

_____

_____

_____

_____

_____

_____

_____

_____

_____

_____

53

Be careful not to go against your creative
vision to fit into someone else's views.

Revise Your Plan

_____

_____

_____

_____

_____

_____

_____

_____

_____

_____

54

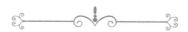

Distractions are one thing but giving up is something else.

Revise Your Plan

_____

_____

_____

_____

_____

_____

_____

_____

_____

_____

55

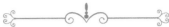

The current version of you should be
setting the table for the future you.

Revise Your Plan

_____

_____

_____

_____

_____

_____

_____

_____

_____

_____

56

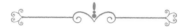

Push away all of your regrets and
pull in all of your potential.

Revise Your Plan

_____

_____

_____

_____

_____

_____

_____

_____

_____

_____

57

Your history will play a major part in your future.

Revise Your Plan

_____

_____

_____

_____

_____

_____

_____

_____

_____

_____

58

Things can happen that can change the way that
you are able to grow but you can activate something
that will allow you to continue growing.

Revise Your Plan

_____

_____

_____

_____

_____

_____

_____

_____

_____

_____

59

Your dreams will kick things off but you
have to take it to the finish line.

Revise Your Plan

_____

_____

_____

_____

_____

_____

_____

_____

_____

_____

60

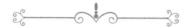

Every now and then you should stop and
admire the new and evolved you.

Revise Your Plan

_____

_____

_____

_____

_____

_____

_____

_____

_____

_____

61

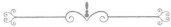

Things will go smoother once you find your groove.

Revise Your Plan

_____

_____

_____

_____

_____

_____

_____

_____

_____

_____

62

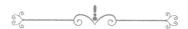

Hang in there as you are being prepped for
your next stage of development.

Revise Your Plan

_____

_____

_____

_____

_____

_____

_____

_____

_____

_____

63

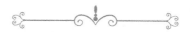

Be more interested in what you can do for yourself more
so that what someone has claimed they will do for you.

Revise Your Plan

_____

_____

_____

_____

_____

_____

_____

_____

_____

64

You really can have many of the things that you envisioned.

Revise Your Plan

_____

_____

_____

_____

_____

_____

_____

_____

_____

65

When people do not allow you into their gatherings you can see it as jacked up or just fine and march on in spite of.

Revise Your Plan

_____

_____

_____

_____

_____

_____

_____

_____

_____

66

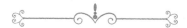

Being redirected can be rewarding.

Revise Your Plan

_____

_____

_____

_____

_____

_____

_____

_____

_____

67

It is time to rebuild what the big bad wolf blew down.

Revise Your Plan

_____

_____

_____

_____

_____

_____

_____

_____

_____

_____

_____

68

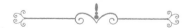

Replenish your heart with all of the good things
that you can recall and move forward.

Revise Your Plan

_____

_____

_____

_____

_____

_____

_____

_____

_____

_____

69

Make choices that can give you a better chance
of obtaining the best outcome for you.

Revise Your Plan

_____

_____

_____

_____

_____

_____

_____

_____

_____

_____

70

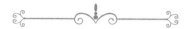

It is time to get serious about who you are!

Revise Your Plan

_____

_____

_____

_____

_____

_____

_____

_____

_____

_____

71

You may not always get paid for the gifts that you provide but it will eventually pay off for you.

Revise Your Plan

_____

_____

_____

_____

_____

_____

_____

_____

_____

_____

72

If you cannot meet your goal in one way
create another way to meet it.

Revise Your Plan

_____

_____

_____

_____

_____

_____

_____

_____

_____

73

Get involved in things that cause you to flourish.

Revise Your Plan

_____

_____

_____

_____

_____

_____

_____

_____

_____

_____

74

When you feel lost just take a little time to revise your thoughts, reroute your steps and move forward.

Revise Your Plan

_____

_____

_____

_____

_____

_____

_____

_____

_____

_____

75

At times the journey can be annoying but the
outcome will provide for your needs.

Revise Your Plan

_____

_____

_____

_____

_____

_____

_____

_____

_____

_____

76

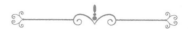

Once you reach your goal prepare to reach another one.

Revise Your Plan

77

When it seems like you are not winning pay attention
to what may be happening to cause those beliefs.

Revise Your Plan

_____

_____

_____

_____

_____

_____

_____

_____

_____

_____

78

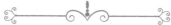

Aim at the things that you want and watch
how many other things fall in place.

Revise Your Plan

_____

_____

_____

_____

_____

_____

_____

_____

_____

_____

79

If you rather fit in opposed to standing out
then you may miss your target.

Revise Your Plan

_____

_____

_____

_____

_____

_____

_____

_____

_____

80

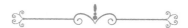

You can have another chance if you set
yourself up for another chance.

Revise Your Plan

_____

_____

_____

_____

_____

_____

_____

_____

_____

81

Do not grow tired of the efforts needed
in order for you to win.

Revise Your Plan

_____

_____

_____

_____

_____

_____

_____

_____

_____

82

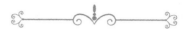

They do not need to be in your circle when you cannot trust them to be in your corner.

Revise Your Plan

_____

_____

_____

_____

_____

_____

_____

_____

_____

_____

83

Changing your route will not be so difficult when you notice that you cannot see the path that you need.

Revise Your Plan

_____

_____

_____

_____

_____

_____

_____

_____

_____

84

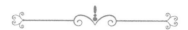

You can make it through this just like
you made it through other things.

Revise Your Plan

_____

_____

_____

_____

_____

_____

_____

_____

_____

85

You have enough evidence that your gifts can
be transferred and used in many ways.

Revise Your Plan

_____

_____

_____

_____

_____

_____

_____

_____

_____

86

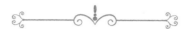

Pay less attention to how long it will take just keep going.

Revise Your Plan

_____

_____

_____

_____

_____

_____

_____

_____

_____

87

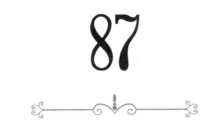

Do not bond with things that are not
compatible with your works.

Revise Your Plan

_____

_____

_____

_____

_____

_____

_____

_____

_____

_____

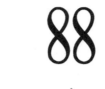

88

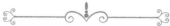

Flip the script on those who said that
things will not work out for you.

Revise Your Plan

_____

_____

_____

_____

_____

_____

_____

_____

_____

_____

89

Give yourself the grace and patience that
you deserve while taking this journey.

Revise Your Plan

_____

_____

_____

_____

_____

_____

_____

_____

_____

_____

90

Bond with those things that contributes to your well-being.

Revise Your Plan

_____

_____

_____

_____

_____

_____

_____

_____

_____

_____

91

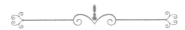

It may bother you but it is alright if certain people are not supporting you while you are in route to your success story.

Revise Your Plan

_____

_____

_____

_____

_____

_____

_____

_____

_____

_____

92

Be careful about who you are seeking attention from.

Revise Your Plan

93

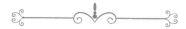

You have the capacity to revise your
setting and defeat your obstacles.

Revise Your Plan

_____

_____

_____

_____

_____

_____

_____

_____

_____

_____

94

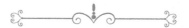

Your spirit will tell you when to transfer
your gifts to another area.

Revise Your Plan

95

Go against the actions that try to stand in your way.

Revise Your Plan

_____

_____

_____

_____

_____

_____

_____

_____

_____

_____

96

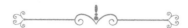

You do not have to push your goals away just because an entity has pushed you away.

Revise Your Plan

_____

_____

_____

_____

_____

_____

_____

_____

_____

_____

97

Schedule an appointment with your true self and do not cancel it even if you find yourself running a little late. You need time to connect with yourself.

Revise Your Plan

_____

_____

_____

_____

_____

_____

_____

_____

_____

_____

98

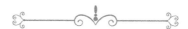

Go after the highest possibility that you have been shown.

Revise Your Plan

_____

_____

_____

_____

_____

_____

_____

_____

_____

_____

99

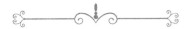

It is one thing to be able to take your gifts
somewhere but it is brave to actually do it.

Revise Your Plan

_____

_____

_____

_____

_____

_____

_____

_____

_____

_____

100

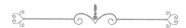

You can change your mind about using your gifts but you cannot change the fact that you have them.

Revise Your Plan

_____

_____

_____

_____

_____

_____

_____

_____

_____

_____

101

You do not have to accept what is being offered
especially if it will steal your authenticity.

Revise Your Plan

_____

_____

_____

_____

_____

_____

_____

_____

_____

_____

102

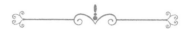

The brush-off that you might receive will not take you
down unless you authorize that downward movement.

Revise Your Plan

103

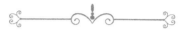

The love and respect that you want can be
quince by showing those things to yourself.

Revise Your Plan

_____

_____

_____

_____

_____

_____

_____

_____

_____

_____

_____

104

Take a chance.

Revise Your Plan

_____

_____

_____

_____

_____

_____

_____

_____

_____

_____

105

If you have done your best keep your chin up.

Revise Your Plan

_____

_____

_____

_____

_____

_____

_____

_____

_____

_____

106

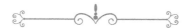

Keep investing in your gifts and plans
and it will take you higher.

Revise Your Plan

_____

_____

_____

_____

_____

_____

_____

_____

_____

107

When you are being redirected to a more suitable
place for your gifts and plans embrace it.

Revise Your Plan

_____

_____

_____

_____

_____

_____

_____

_____

_____

_____

Remember to replenish your heart with all of the good things that you can recall and move forward in a positive way. You are definitely worth it.

Printed in the United States
by Baker & Taylor Publisher Services